Insightful Self-Therapy

Increasing Your Awareness about
Mental Health and
How to Live a Happier Life

Bardolf & Company

INSIGHTFUL SELF-THERAPY
Increasing Your Awareness about Mental Health and
How to Live a Happier Life

ISBN 978-1-938842-61-0
Copyright © 2023 by Denise Schonwald

Published by Bardolf & Company
www.bardolfandcompany.com

Cover design by *shawcreativegroup.com*
Erica Ellis, Ink Deep Editing
Christine Nicole of Portrait Boutique
    for pictures of Denise and Henry

This book is dedicated to all of you
who invest in your mental health
for the benefit of your family, yourselves,
and everyone you meet.
May others feel the Divine through you,
and may they be blessed by your presence.

I also dedicate this book
to my husband, Harvey,
and the rest of my family and friends,
who are always encouraging me
and challenging me to be better.
They lead by example, and I am grateful
for their leadership and love.
My late parents would be proud knowing
that their daughters are doing their best
to leave the world a better place,
the same as they did for us.

Contents

Insightful Self-Therapy

Increasing Your Awareness about
Mental Health and
How to Live a Happier Life

Denise Schonwald
BSRN, LMHC

Bardolf & Company
Sarasota, Florida

Introduction

I have been practicing as either a nurse or a therapist for over thirty years. My first career was as a critical care nurse, a profession I loved dearly. A decade ago, I decided to go back to school to become a mental health counselor and have been working in private practice ever since. Over the years, I have been able to combine my training and expertise in both medicine and psychology to help my clients live healthier lives physically, emotionally, and spiritually. My first book, *Healing Your Body By Mastering Your Mind*, helped readers learn how their mental health is connected to their physical health. It was well received, and many felt it gave them added insight into how the body communicates and how they can take a more active role in their own health and well-being.

Today, many people are busy and feel they have little time to read a lengthy book or to listen to a podcast for more than thirty minutes. When I decided to start writing my second book, *Insightful Self-Therapy*, I wanted to create a short yet powerful read to include those "on the go" individuals, providing some "food for thought" and helpful tips. Over the years, I have found short quick reads to be the most powerful and effective. This read is similar to a daily devotional but it is geared toward mental health. It should be digested one chapter at a time, as it may be more helpful if you take in a small amount of information in one sitting. It can also serve as a reference book to refer back to from time to time.

I am sad to say that most people neglect their mental health. The day-to-day stress of managing bills, family, work, and other obligations often leaves little time to care for ourselves. Yet our mental health is the key to optimal physical health, happy relationships, and overall feelings of peace and happiness. Ultimately, addressing our own needs reflects the value we place on ourselves. *Insightful Self-Therapy* will teach you about everyday problems many of us face and provide helpful tools for correcting them.

I hope you enjoy this book and that it offers you insight and healing. I am available for speaking engagements, counseling, and performing psychological evaluations nationally. Please feel free to visit me on my website to learn more at *deniseschonwald.com*. Self-scheduling makes booking an appointment quick and easy. I am looking forward to hearing from you.

Denise Schonwald
May 2023

Chapter 1

Quiz:

Understanding Your Mental Health

Let's get started. How well do you know your mental health? Take the quiz and find out. Pick one of the five answers for each question below:

When it comes to your mindset about yourself, your needs and desires, what best describes you?

1. There are many ways I am practicing a life of abundance, happiness, and joy.

2. There are opportunities and possibilities to make my life even better than it is now.

3. I just want to try and get through this week, month, or year.

4. I try not to even think about it.

5. I feel guilty putting myself first.

When it comes to knowing what you really want in your life, you feel as if:

1. I have spent a lot of time reflecting on my beliefs, values, and the other important aspects of my life.

2. I know what I want in some areas but would like to gain greater awareness in other areas.

3. I don't know what I want or need just yet.

4. I feel completely overwhelmed just thinking about it.

5. I have no idea how to answer this question.

When it comes to having a positive and mindful self-care routine:

1. Every day is filled with joy, peace, and gratefulness.
2. I feel a sense of adequacy and am generally content.
3. I have good days but they aren't as consistent as I want them to be
4. I wonder how I will ever find time to add myself to my already hectic life.
5. I am worried about my health and my emotional well-being, and I am exhausted most of the time.

When it comes to spirituality:

1. I am clear on what spirituality means to me and it is a big part of my life.
2. I grew up learning about God and religion, but I no longer connect with it.
3. I would say I'm spiritual and believe in God, but I don't really practice spirituality.
4. I have no idea what practicing spirituality even means.
5. I don't feel that spirituality or faith have anything to do with physical and emotional health, but I am open to learning more.

When it comes to having a plan for yourself and taking action:

1. I have a number of mindful healthy practices and cannot imagine living my life without them because they are a part of who I am.
2. I try to make time for myself but it is rare.
3. I know it is important to take time for myself but I have no idea what to do.
4. I start taking action, feel better, and then stop.
5. I feel selfish when I make time for myself.

Score results:

1 = 5 points
2 = 4 points
3 = 3 points
4 = 2 points
5 = 1 point

Score of 20-25: You rock! You most definitely have learned a lot about mindfulness and self-awareness, and you are making the world a better place by taking care of yourself. Your positive energy has a ripple effect, and I would love to help you continue your journey.

15-19: You are on your way! You have scratched the surface and are learning. I applaud you for starting to take care of you.

10-14: You have walked over to a very large pool, but you have only dipped your toe in. You have started to build some awareness of how to live a happier, healthier, and abundant life. Keep going!

5-9: If you want to stay healthy, you may want to take a hard look at your habits and practices.

1-5: You are at risk for emotional instability and physical illness. The body follows the mind.

The secret to having it all is knowing you already do.

Take a moment and think about this, maybe even close your eyes. When you invest in yourself, everyone around you benefits: your partner, your children, your siblings, your coworkers, your neighbors, everyone you meet. Never underestimate the power of your ripple.

Keep your results and responses in mind while you're reading. If you want to talk more about your own mental health and how you can improve it, please make an appointment to meet with me. One of the best gifts you can give yourself is the gift of healing.

We all have an inner knowing,
but we pretend that we don't.

—Author unknown

Chapter 2

Why Do We Ignore Our Mental Health

Every day, we are reminded how important it is to take care of our physical health. From diet to exercise and sleep, everyone understands that taking care of our bodies is necessary for optimal health—even if we don't always follow the best practices to achieve that goal. However, our mental health, though arguably as important to our quality of life, is rarely discussed. In fact, many of us hide the fact that we are experiencing anxiety or depression, or feeling overwhelmed. We've not been taught to prioritize mental health. Because of that, some people may even feel shame about their emotions.

I have found it often takes a trip or two to the emergency room and a diagnosis of a panic attack to convince a person they need help managing their anxiety. In the mental health profession, we are seeing an increased number of clients coming in for the first visit with a decade or more history of depression. Many times, trauma or a difficult childhood were contributing factors. I'm sad to say the suicide rate is higher than ever. I was recently told the leading cause of death of police officers is suicide.

Psychologically Speaking

Most people delay getting help because they feel their struggles are just a part of life they need to deal with. Many people pack their schedules full so they stay busy enough to push anxious and depressive thoughts to the back of their minds.

Others feel counseling is not worth the price. It is disheartening that a lot of people think getting their hair colored or buying a purse is a better use of their money than helping themselves mentally.

Today, the stigma of going to counseling is lifting. I have heard people say, "You only go to counseling when you're crazy," but the truth is you should go to counseling when you don't know what to do in order to feel peace, happiness, and fulfillment. Every developmental stage we go through will cause the body to struggle. It is much easier to correct irrational thinking and behaviors sooner rather than later.

Call to Action

I created a poster to be displayed in hallways and break rooms in the workplace, which I have included below. I donate these posters to the police department, fire department, schools, hospitals, and anyone else who would like one. The message is simple but powerful, and I hope you can incorporate these suggestions into your own life.

MENTAL HEALTH

THE BEST PROTECTION YOU CAN HAVE ON THE JOB

MAKE time for self care (hobbies)

EXERCISE regularly to balance brain chemestry

NUTRITION- Eating regular healthy meals to fuel the mind & body

TRAIN your mind to refrain from negativity

AVOID harmful habits to relieve tension such as smoking, alcohol, gambling, etc.

LAUGH often and connect with friends

HIGHER POWER: connection to God or the Universe through prayer or meditation

EXPLORE opportunites for personal growth (podcasts, books, classes)

ALLOW the body the rest it requires

LEARN to recognize your body's response to stress (overeaating, irritaability, exhaustion)

TALK & communicate openly with friends & family

HELP is available and not a sign of weakness

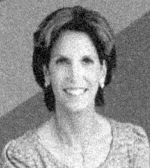

Denise Schonwald, BSRN, LMHC
Nationally Licensed Mental Health Counselor
w w w.deniseschonwald.com

There is a Divine source. When you recognize it, acknowledge it, and surrender to it, you won't have to suffer.

—*Iyanla Van Zant*

Chapter 3

Spirituality and Mental Health

Most people use the terms "religion" and "spirituality" interchangeably, as they both hold the promise of comfort and peace in an uncertain world. But although the two concepts may seem similar, they are quite different.

Spirituality strives to understand a human's connection to the world and each other. Religion is more structured and organized, with guidelines representing community members' beliefs and worldviews. Since both spirituality and religion can inspire peace, comfort, and strength, people often fall back on their spiritual or religious beliefs to endure challenging situations. Holding to a belief system is a significant factor in improving one's mental health and well-being.

Some of the benefits of seeking a spiritual life include:

1. **Develops a sense of community:** Individuals often create a community with people with similar spiritual or religious belief systems. This can provide support,

social interaction, and trustworthy relationships that can significantly reinforce individual mental health.

2. **Strengthens self-esteem:** Spirituality provides feelings of self-empowerment, strengthening our belief system while accepting other people regardless of their individual religious and spiritual beliefs.

3. **Inspires mindfulness:** Spirituality is associated with meditation and self-reflection, healthy practices that positively impact an individual's mental state.

4. **Establishes unity with their environment:** Spiritual and religious teachings emphasize being mindful of personal actions and doing the right thing. They teach forgiveness, compassion, and gratitude—all of which help people weather difficult seasons of life.

5. **Calms the mind:** Spirituality can significantly influence the creation of calm and serenity as well as reduce stress and anxiety. Religious rituals or practices establish structure, predictability, and consistency—solid ground for people undergoing difficult circumstances.

Psychologically Speaking

Cynics may not see the connection between spirituality and mental well-being. And it is true that religion and spirituality are often used as a superficial Band-Aid and can make people feel worse. When someone genuinely seeks a solution to a profound life issue, being dismissed with sentiments like "You just need to have more faith" can be harmful. But many spiritual disciplines can—and do—improve mental health for millions of believers. Faith and spirituality are powerful when combined with compassion, openness, and positivity. When we are going through rough times, we have an opportunity to strengthen our belief in God, which can deepen our sense of purpose. A therapist can also help. When looking for a therapist, particularly one who incorporates spirituality or religious faith, make sure they are properly trained and educated. There are numerous programs available today offering certifications in counseling and coaching but, unfortunately, some of these programs offer minimal training.

Call to Action

Practicing spirituality is like exercising a muscle. You need to make it a daily practice. I recommend starting your day with a fifteen- to twenty-minute meditation. When you first wake up, go to the bathroom and then get back into bed. Close your eyes and allow your mind to relax, which will be easier since you have not yet awakened fully. Take a few deep breaths and practice gratitude. Ask God or the Universe to connect to you throughout the day through your intuition, synchronicities, and your experiences with others. Envision your perfect day and review your goals for yourself short term, within the year, and long term. Say a blessing for others and then for yourself. Open your eyes, take another deep breath, and start your day.

You don't have to see the whole staircase, just take the first step.

—*Martin Luther King Jr.*

Chapter 4

Anxiety and Stress

When we experience a frightening, stressful, or even unfamiliar situation, the mind and body often react with anxious emotions. This may be a general sense of uneasiness or a feeling of outright distress or dread. Some level of anxiety is our mind's method of staying alert and aware, but those with anxiety disorders can feel debilitated and unable to function. When we experience things that happen in our world, outside of our bodies, the body relies on the mind to interpret it. This is what we call perception. One person may perceive a house full of company as joyful, while another person might perceive the same experience as stressful and overwhelming. In general, happy people practice mindfulness (noticing and awareness) of how they perceive situations, while anxious people have a tendency to look at the events and experiences of their lives through a lens of fear. The body can't tell the difference between what is real and what is imagined, which is why some people can have a panic attack grocery shopping with no one around.

When the mind is not healthy, an individual will lead with phrases like "I'm nervous about," "I'm worried because," "I'm scared because," which will automatically cause the body to express a stress response.

Psychologically speaking:

Anxiety, to put it simply, is "fake" fear. As I mentioned, our minds act as translators to our body. When the body receives information from the mind, it will respond accordingly. Anxious thinking will eventually manifest physically: heart and lung problems, stomach issues, breast cancer—the list is extensive. Psychologically, when a person is fearful about almost everything, the ability to discern what is truly concerning gets skewed. I have seen many anxious clients overlook dangerous circumstances because they have lost their ability to clearly evaluate a situation logically and appropriately.

Call to Action:

Practice reframing and interpreting situations more positively. If you are a "stinking thinking" kind of person, this may be a tough job for you. For example, you have received a "C" on a test, and you're catastrophizing by saying "I just got a 'C' on my exam and now I'll never graduate, get a good job, or be able to support myself." Instead, say "I studied hard for my test. I hope I can learn from my mistakes and study more efficiently next time." OR "I didn't really study as much as I should have, and I am not going to be able to get a better grade unless I put in the study time." You can reframe any situation, no matter how difficult. A therapist can help.

Eating to turn off feelings doesn't
fully appease your feeling; instead
it just adds more psychological and
caloric weight to the experience.

—*Jennifer L. Taiez*

Chapter 5

Overeating

Eating is something we all need to do every day to supply our bodies with the nutrition they need to stay healthy. Yet, when we start to use food to help us cope with emotions, such as low self-worth, fear, lack of trust, and overthinking, it can quickly lead to other problems.

Nearly everyone will overeat sometimes, whether it be a special occasion or a lazy day at home. But when overeating becomes a habit or is connected to other disorders, there may be a reason for concern. Whether we realize it or not, we all have some form of "relationship" with food, which is typically driven by emotion. In fact, emotions are the underlying cause of eating disorders, and debilitating shame and guilt are often the result. The good news is that, with some effort, you can improve your eating habits and take control of your emotional and mental health.

Psychologically Speaking

Overeating is a symptom indicating the body needs ease. Eating can relieve anxiety and depression, and is often one of the first indicators of these types of issues.

Indications you may have an overeating problem:
An inability to stop eating and a disinterest in doing so

- Rapidly and repeatedly ingesting significant amounts of food
- Continuing to consume food after feeling full
- Never feeling emotional or physical satisfaction
- Constantly feeling apathy and emotional numbness
- Feeling guilt and worthlessness connected to the behavior

Many people look for the "quick fix," which is why the diet industry has been so lucrative. While certain diets do work and people can lose weight, they frequently gain the weight right back when they go off the diet, sometimes gaining back even more than they lost. Years ago, I gave a lecture called "It's not what you're eating, but what's eating you" to help people learn that overeating has a root emotional cause. If this cause is not treated, no diet or surgery will be successful.

Call to Action

If you engage in overeating or binge eating, seek professional help to face these issues effectively. A mental health counselor can help you discover the root causes of both conditions and work with you to develop a plan for facing them. Your mental health is just as essential as your physical health, so don't delay in getting help.

A licensed therapist is instrumental in identifying destructive weight-control behaviors such as:

- Nutritional constraints and phobias
- Purging behaviors

- Unhealthy body avoidance and negative self-image
- Self-worth and self-esteem issues

When addressing negative overeating habits, it is important to understand how depression and low self-esteem issues are at play. Overeating and weight gain can further impact how you view yourself. Instead of hoping willpower and self-restricting rules do the trick, look to a mental health therapist or mindful eating coach to help you regain control of your thoughts, habits, and life.

> True forgiveness is when you can say
> "thank you for that experience."
>
> —*Oprah Winfrey.*

Chapter 6

Forgiveness and Healing: Forgiving Others

We are given the opportunity to forgive people every day. And while we can easily forgive someone who forgot to call us back after a missed phone call or who had to cancel a lunch date, there are some circumstances in life when forgiveness seems impossible. How can you forgive someone who has caused profound damage to your heart, body, or mind?

We are often presented with situations that cause anger, pain, and sorrow, and the hurt feels significantly worse when the person inflicting the pain is close to us. Whether an innocent mistake or a deliberate betrayal, the breach of a close personal relationship can feel devastating and irreparable. Even if we forgive the actual act in question, trust is difficult to reestablish and rebuild.

One of life's most significant challenges is moving on from the pain such a deep wound can cause. But establishing a path toward forgiveness is the key to protecting your physical and mental health. When unforgiveness is allowed to fester, it can cause stress, anxiety, and depression.

The Benefits of Forgiveness

Although forgiveness can be challenging and complex, there is no argument among experts that forgiveness is essential for personal well-being. Cultivating the ability to forgive has substantial benefits, including:

1. **Freedom from the burden:** You may not even realize just how heavy the weight of unforgiveness is until you lay it down. Carrying hurt and resentment can become part of our character, making us cynical and bitter. You end up inflicting more self-harm than you realize.

2. **Improved physical health:** Strange as it may sound, studies have shown that forgiving other people is vital to maintaining optimal physical health, most notably heart health. The ability to forgive and let go of hurt reduces the risk of heart attack, lowers high blood pressure and cholesterol, and even gives us a higher tolerance for physical pain. Deciding to forgive and release anger also results in better sleep, which is essential to physical well-being.

3. **Mental health benefits:** People experience less anxiety and depression when they forgive others, and stress levels tend to be lower across the board.

4. **More genuine relationships:** The more adept we become at forgiving people in our lives, the more our relationships improve and become more genuine. After all, we all make mistakes, and we hope the people we are closest to will forgive us. Having grace for others' mistakes will allow them to have grace for yours.

Psychologically Speaking

Refusing to forgive keeps us trapped in the past and prevents us from enjoying our daily lives. Many of us regret how we've interacted with others and wish we could have done things differently. Just as people have hurt us, we have hurt others. The truth is we are not perfect, and we learn by making mistakes. By understanding this, we can forgive others and also finally forgive ourselves—which may be the most crucial benefit of embracing forgiveness.

The decision to forgive and move on from hurt and disappointment is the first step toward true healing of the heart and mind. Healing is impossible without forgiveness first, as resentment and bitterness cause too much emotional and physical damage—whether or not we are aware of the harm we are inflicting on ourselves.

However, if you have forgiven and were hurt by the same person again, you will need to make a shift in that relationship or perhaps distance yourself from the person. This can be challenging when the person is a family member. In these cases, you may need to adjust the degree of your interactions with them.

Call to Action

Take out a piece of paper and Write down all the people who have hurt you, betrayed you or disappointed you. Next to their name, write down what you are forgiving them for. For example: "Dad — I am forgiving you for not being a better father to me. I realize you were struggling with your own pain and I am no longer going to harbor bitterness and resentment toward you."

I did this a few months ago. At first I couldn't think of anything. But then I started writing. The more I wrote, the more things came up. When you are finished writing, if you want to take this further, tear up the paper(s), put them in a bowl, walk outside, and burn them. As the smoke goes up into the sky, say to yourself, "I release all of this to the Universe, as I no longer wish to hold it." When I did this, it was a very healing exercise, and I think it could be for you too.

> If I am not good to myself, how can I expect someone else to be good to me?
>
> —*Maya Angelou*

Chapter 7

Why It Is Important to Forgive Yourself

Forgiveness is a deliberate decision to release feelings of resentment, anger, and vengeance toward someone who has wronged you. Forgiveness benefits both physical and mental well-being. It can be challenging to release feelings of bitterness and truly forgive. But as hard as forgiving others may be, forgiving ourselves can be significantly more challenging. Self-forgiveness is not about absolving yourself from any mistake or wrongdoing.

Much like forgiving someone else, forgiving yourself involves:

1. **Understanding your feelings and emotions:** Developing an awareness of feelings is essential when learning to forgive yourself. Identifying and naming your emotions often reduces the intensity of related guilt and shame.

2. **Accepting personal responsibility for what occurred:** Rationalizing, justifying, or making excuses for your actions often impairs the forgiveness process. You can prevent negative emotions by accepting responsibility for any actions that have harmed others.

3. **Regarding yourself with compassion:** Learn to offer yourself the same compassion you would extend to someone else. Forgiving yourself means acknowledging that you made a mistake but resolving to do better in the future—and giving yourself a break.

4. **Expressing remorse for your errant words or actions:** When we accept responsibility, we often experience damaging emotions like guilt and shame. Guilt is healthy and understandable when you've done something wrong, but remorse should be used to stimulate a desire to change.

5. **Making amends with all parties and apologizing— even to yourself:** Making amends is an essential aspect of forgiveness, even when the individual you are forgiving is yourself. One way to ease your guilt is to take practical action to right your wrongs, starting with an apology.

6. **Discerning lessons to be learned:** Giving into self-pity or even self-hatred is harmful and makes it nearly impossible to stay positive and motivated. Forgiving yourself means finding the lessons to be learned and allowing yourself to grow from mistakes.

Did You Know? There is a difference between guilt and shame. Experiencing guilt means that you are a good person who did something you regret. Shame, however, implies that you feel you are a terrible person or have a failure of character, which can inspire feelings of worthlessness and lead to addiction, depression, and aggression.

Psychologically Speaking

Forgiving ourselves is a powerful exercise, but it doesn't work for everyone. Those who irrationally blame themselves even when they are not at fault, for instance, may not be able to find a way to forgive themselves. In addition, those who have experienced abuse or trauma may be consumed by shame and guilt about circumstances out of their control.

However, self-forgiveness offers a multitude of benefits.

1. **Mental Health:** Offering forgiveness to yourself enhances self-worth and boosts feelings of wellness. Research has shown that when people practice self-forgiveness, they are less prone to depression and anxiety and enjoy elevated productivity, focus, and concentration levels.

2. **Physical Health:** Forgiveness can also positively influence physical health, such as improving cholesterol levels, reducing pain, lowering blood pressure, and minimizing the chances of a heart attack.

3. **Relationships:** A forgiving and compassionate attitude is critical to enjoying successful relationships. Establishing close emotional bonds with others is essential, but so is the capability to restore those connections when they become damaged.

Call To Action

Write down no more than three things you need to forgive yourself for. Next to each item, write lessons that you learned from these mistakes and ways you grew because of them.

Don't give up because of one bad chapter
in your life. Keep going. Your story doesn't
end here.

—*HealthyPlace.com*

Chapter 8

Situational Depression

There are times in our lives where we feel overwhelmed, sad or even depressed. Certain events that fundamentally change our circumstances are tougher to handle than normal challenges and can plunge us into a season of despair. This psychological reaction is called situational, short-term, or reactive depression. A type of adjustment disorder, it is different from chronic depression because it is caused by a reaction to a certain event. Some examples include:

1. Children going off to college
2. Retiring
3. Moving to a new city or state.
4. Changing jobs
5. Selling the family home in order to downsize
6. Losing our parents
7. Relationship problems
8. Divorce
9. Illness
10. Death of a loved one

When an individual is otherwise mentally healthy, these types of events can cause depressive symptoms. and generally improve in six months. To be clear, this does not mean we forget about what happened and return to normal. Rather, the body and mind find a "new" normal or simply adjust to new circumstances and adapt. Some of the symptoms of situational depression are:

1. Trouble sleeping (insomnia)
2. Excessive worrying (anxiety)
3. Fatigue
4. Decreased or increased appetite
5. Feeling hopeless or crying easily
6. Isolating oneself from others
7. Loss of interest in things you used to enjoy
8. Difficulty concentrating and doing things that used to be routine.

Psychologically Speaking

Every stage of our development has its own set of challenges. For example, most people think retirement, traditionally called the "golden years," should be a time when we're happy and joyful because we have worked all our lives and can now relax. Yet, our identity for decades has been connected to our profession. While we know we need to do something else with our time, it can be difficult to reinvent ourselves. We now have a lot more free time, nowhere to be and no one to report to. This can be both exciting and unnerving at the same time.

If we all of a sudden find ourselves divorced after decades of marriage, how do we manage that? Even though we might feel relieved, because we are "free" and out of an unhappy marriage, the thought of moving forward on our own might feel overwhelming and scary. Some of my clients in this situation are in their 60s and 70s but haven't been on their own since their 20s or maybe ever! That can be a difficult period of adjustment, and depression can be a phase.

Call to Action

First of all, there is nothing wrong with you. Nor are you weak or incapable. You are struggling after a stressful event that has happened in your life. It doesn't matter what the event is, whether it be the death of a spouse or the death of a pet, you are suffering. Here are a few ways to help you through tough times:

1. Lean on friends and family who are supportive of you.
2. If you are religious, rely on your church, mosque or synagogue for help.
3. Consider seeking professional counseling even if it is short term.
4. Make time for self-care and be compassionate with yourself.
5. Take naps if you feel tired.
6. Hydrate and eat balanced meals.
7. Avoid drinking too much alcohol or use of other substances.
8. If your symptoms are not alleviating, consult your doctor.

If your depression lingers and won't go away, it may be time to consult with a professional counselor or therapist (see next chapter).

Depression is being colorblind and
constantly told how colorful the world is.

—*Atticus Poetry*

Chapter 9

Chronic Depression

Depression is prevalent in our society. Unfortunately, many people struggle with depressive symptoms to the point where it becomes part of their everyday life. Clinical depression is a diagnosed condition that can be crippling and life-altering. A person suffering from clinical depression may have trouble getting out of bed, bathing, brushing their teeth, or even eating. When a person becomes clinically depressed, medical intervention or hospitalization is usually necessary. However, other forms of depression can be left unaddressed. Because the word "depression" can refer to both a clinical condition and an emotional episode, it can easily be misunderstood. There are many different types of depression that we will explore here together.

Psychologically Speaking

Depression is a mood disorder causing persistent feelings of sadness. It is often accompanied by an intense apathy towards people and activities that typically provide joy and meaning. Depression impacts how the individual feels, thinks, and behaves, and often significantly inhibits a person's ability to function effectively.

There are many types of depression, and many different things cause depressive emotions. Here are five of the most common forms of depression we see in society.

1. Major Depressive Disorder: The term "clinical depression" refers to major depressive disorder. Those with major depressive disorder exhibit several key traits: depressed mood, apathy, weight changes, sleep changes, fatigue, feelings of worthlessness and guilt, lack of focus, and suicidal tendencies.

   If these symptoms are present for longer than two weeks, they will often receive a diagnosis of major depressive disorder.

2. Persistent Depressive Disorder: In recent years, a condition called dysthymia has been renamed persistent depressive disorder. Persistent depressive disorder is a form of chronic depression that frequently manifests over two years. Persistent depressive disorder symptoms can be mild, moderate, or severe. There may be short periods when the depression lifts, but this relief typically only lasts several weeks. While not considered as serious as major depressive disorder, symptoms are evasive and enduring. These symptoms may include sadness, loss of pleasure, anger, irritability, guilt, low self-esteem, insomnia, oversleeping, loss of appetite, hopelessness, and loss of focus.

3. Bipolar Disorder: Bipolar disorder is characterized by periods of mania, an abnormally elevated mood. These periods of mania may be mild, or they can be so severe as to cause significant life impairment, necessitate hospitalization, or influence a person's perception of reality. Most individuals diagnosed with bipolar disorder also experience major depressive episodes. Bipolar individuals exhibit all the signs of depression mentioned above, as well as lethargy,

unexplained pain, indecision, and disorganization. In extreme cases, psychosis and hallucination may occur, and the risk of suicide is high.

4. Postpartum Depression: Pregnancy often causes hormonal swings that affect mood. This type of depression can first manifest during pregnancy or following the child's birth. More than just "baby blues," postpartum depression causes mood swings, anxiety, and irritability. Postpartum depression typically lasts about two weeks, but severe cases have been known to persist much longer. In addition to intense mood swings, symptoms may include sadness, social isolation, trouble bonding with the infant, loss of appetite, hopelessness, feeling inadequate, experiencing panic or anxiety attacks, and thoughts of self-harm (or harm to the baby.) Left untreated, postpartum depression may last as long as a year, but antidepressants, counseling, and hormone therapy have proven to be effective treatments.

5. Atypical Depression: As its name indicates, this disorder does not follow the standard progression and presentation of other common forms of depression. People with atypical depression may experience excessive eating or weight gain, excessive sleep, fatigue or weakness, sensitivity to rejection, and disproportionate adverse reactions. However, these individuals typically "bounce back" quickly when circumstances change, they get good news, or a problem resolves.

Call to Action:

To adequately treat depression, you must determine exactly what you are facing. If your medical doctor cannot isolate a physical reason for your symptoms, call a certified mental health counselor to get the help you need.

Parents love their children unconditionally
and applaud them wholeheartedly when
they actually take the risk to make
a difference for the good in their own life
and in the world.

—*Breaking the Trance*
by George Lynn and Cynthia Johnson.

Chapter 10

Parenting

Being a parent is an extremely rewarding journey, but it does not come without its struggles, trials, and tribulations. Children are constantly sending us signals, and sometimes those signals are difficult to read. Are they hungry? Tired? Angry? And the signals from one child won't necessarily be the same as the signals from your other children. That's the one sure thing about parenting—every child is different and has different ways of interacting with the environment, their friends, and their families.

Sometimes your child will go through a rough patch and will act out in destructive or unacceptable ways (screaming, throwing objects, the works). When your child is acting out or having an emotional meltdown, it can be very difficult to keep your cool and keep your own emotions under control.

Parenting support or counseling can be helpful for parents of children of any age, from infants to teenagers. It can help you through many of the tough decisions that you will face in parenthood, including those regarding setting expectations, proper discipline, and finding a balance between being a parent and empowering yourself.

Many parents think meeting with a parenting counselor is a sign of weakness or failure, but this is far from the truth. Parenting is an extremely important responsibility, and it should provide joy and gratification as part of the human journey.

Psychologically Speaking

Structure and guidance are extremely important for children, and if not provided, it can have long-term effects on their well-being. Personality disorders such as borderline personality disorder, obsessive compulsive disorder, and narcissistic personality disorder can cause even more challenges later on when these children enter adulthood.

A few tips to help children thrive:

1. Provide structure and stability. Going to sleep at a regular bedtime, following household rules and boundaries, and completing chores help children gain confidence and develop good habits.

2. Eat together. It might be surprising to know that many families today do not eat any meals together. With busy work and school schedules, breakfast and lunch might be impossible to coordinate. However, dinner time is an excellent time to break bread together, enjoy each other's company, and share your day with each other. It is also a good time for children to learn good table manners and social etiquette. Limit screen time. Research has shown that too much screen time is harmful to both mental and physical health. Adverse effects include anger issues, emotional instability, fatigue, and neurological tics in some instances.

3. Provide stability. Children need to grow up in a home with emotionally stable parents. Addictions,

anger management issues, and marital strife can cause children to feel unprotected and insecure. Parents need to take responsibility for their own mental health. Counseling may be helpful.

Call to Action

Here are a few steps for parents to start doing today:

Monitor your own screen time. Lead by example and model the behaviors you want to see in your children.

1. Take care of your own physical and mental health. Eat balanced meals, drink plenty of water, and eliminate sodas and junk food.

2. Speak clearly and set boundaries with children. Don't resort to screaming to show you're serious and want your children to do something.

3. Enforce consequences but not with bitterness and resentment.

4. Always speak calmly. Our words are a lot more effective when we speak with self-control, grace, and dignity.

He who blames others has a long way
to go on his journey. He who blames
himself is halfway there. He who
blames no one has arrived.

—*Chinese proverb*

Chapter 11

Helping Children Through Divorce

A divorce is one of the most emotionally challenging events many experience, affecting all areas of life and many relationships beyond the divorcing couple. In many cases, parents, siblings, and friends struggle with feelings of sadness, anger, and confusion—while also trying to navigate the perceived need to choose sides. But no one is more affected by the pain of divorce than the children involved, who may suffer various psychological effects. Their reactions, emotions, and even trauma shape their childhood and often follow them into adulthood and color their own relationships.

A common belief is that children are resilient and able to adapt to the situation, which is true in many cases. But while a parental divorce is stressful for all children, some kids heal and recover better than others. It is essential for parents to proactively take steps to minimize the detrimental effects of their divorce on their children.

There are many ways for parents to help reduce their children's negative emotions:

1. **Practice Peaceful Co-Parenting:** Constant conflict, especially overt hostility and fighting between their parents, increases stress in children and has been linked to negative behavioral issues. But children also sense and react to minor tension, making it necessary for divorcing couples to interact peacefully and in a friendly manner. If you cannot accomplish this, seek professional help, as it is vital for your child's emotional health.

2. **Help Kids Feel Safe:** When one parent leaves, a child can experience intense feelings of abandonment and anxiety. It can make them fear the future and can affect their self-esteem. Helping your children feel secure and loved will help alleviate their fears and reduce the risks of future mental health issues.

3. **Don't Put Children in the Middle:** Divorcing couples often put their children in the middle of their conflict, asking them to relay messages or inquiring if the other parent is dating. This behavior is inappropriate and places undue pressure and anxiety on the children. Parents should never discuss the other parent unless it is on favorable terms. The children should never be asked to choose a side or express "whom they like better"—nor be expected to listen to complaints about a parent they love.

4. **Practice Consistent Discipline:** After a divorce, one parent may strive to be more lenient to keep the children happy. However, different levels of discipline are detrimental to a child's growth and can cause them to exploit the situation. Parents need to agree on appropriate rules and established consequences,

which research has shown reduces behavioral issues and delinquency as children grow.

5. **Keep an Eye on Teenagers:** When children become adolescents and are out of the house more often, their emotions and suppressed feelings about the divorce can result in behavioral problems. These issues can be far more dangerous than with younger kids and can include substance abuse or other risky behaviors. Keeping the lines of communication open, maintaining a loving relationship, and intervening at the first sign of a problem are key.

Psychologically Speaking

During my years of practice, I have seen many children who were struggling as a result of their parents' divorce. Unfortunately, the hurt and frustration from a crumbling marriage can sometimes be projected onto the children. We talked about this already, but it is important to reiterate. When couples divorce cooperatively, making a conscious effort to protect their children's well-being, the children are able to heal and lead healthy lives. Tension, aggression, and modeling poor behavior in front of children can have lasting effects on them and may lead to personality disorders or chronic health problems in severe cases.

There are other stressors many children face when their parents divorce. In most instances, children will split their time 50/50 between Mom's house and Dad's house. This, alone, can be very challenging, as they have to live between two homes, two sets of rules, two different beds to sleep on, etc. It can be worth the investment for the children to have a fairly full wardrobe in both homes. Parents should do their best to help their children adapt, while offering compassion, love, and support along the way.

Call to Action

Write down thoughts and ideas about how you can avoid making your children take sides so you are prepared. And be willing to compromise and negotiate with your ex. This doesn't mean you should always give in. It simply means you are willing to put your own needs and wants aside for the sake of the children. For example, your holiday is Christmas Day and your family lives locally. Your ex's family will be visiting from out of town, and they would like to take the children on Christmas Day so they can watch them open presents. Perhaps you could have your family over on a different day to celebrate Christmas, especially since your family lives near you. Compromising doesn't make you weak; it makes you a stronger team player, which is really all that matters when it comes to your children.

Disciplining yourself to do what you know is right and important, although difficult, is the high road to pride, self-esteem, and personal satisfaction.

—*Margaret Thatcher*

Chapter 12

Self-Worth and Self-Esteem

Self-worth and self-esteem refer to the value we place on ourselves. It is an internal sense of feeling worthy of love. When we think about interactions and relationships with our friends, family, coworkers, and neighbors, we emphasize concepts such as kindness, consideration, respect, love, and affirmation. However, many people don't apply those ideas to their own self-image. The extent to which we consider ourselves worthy of those same ideals determines our level of self-worth and/or self-esteem.

Low self-image can be linked to depression and anxiety. Individuals who don't have a sense of worth may be irritable and anxious, and often experience fatigue, weight issues, insomnia, and lack of focus. They may also:

- have a negative view of themselves
- lack trust in their own capabilities
- have a constant fear of failure

- focus disproportionately on their failures and weaknesses
- struggle with accepting compliments or praise
- put others on pedestals they may not deserve
- minimize their own needs
- constantly compare themselves with others
- allow personal boundaries to be violated
- try to gain acceptance by people-pleasing
- rarely defend themselves

Psychologically Speaking

One of the contributing factors to low self-worth is negative self-talk. Starting a sentence with "I'm so stupid, I never realized..." or "I'm so pathetic, I can't believe I didn't..." isn't helpful. I would hope no one would speak to another person that way, and they shouldn't speak to themselves like that either.

When people with low self-worth make small mistakes or poor decisions, it only adds to the layers of shame and guilt they hold inside of themselves. One simple practice to help with low self-worth is to learn ways to process events, decisions, and choices more positively. Another is to spend an hour each day working on your personal growth. This can be in the form of reading self-help books, listening to podcasts on self-esteem, journaling, meditating or any other form of self-care. It could be a walk, a bath, or even a massage. This sounds fairly easy to do and even pleasurable but the majority of clients I see suffering from low self-worth have difficulty following through with these fairly simple suggestions.

Call to Action

Here are a few ways you can improve your self-esteem:

Challenge Yourself through Exercise: Studies prove that exercise is associated with higher self-worth. Challenging your body and working toward goals provides tangible proof that you are capable of more than you imagined. Not only that, but exercise provides a wealth of physical and mental benefits.

Spend Time Doing Things You Are Good At: Finding something you love and are good at reinforces confidence. Teaching others your skill—be it musical, artistic, mechanical, or creative—can boost your mood and allow you to show off your proficiency.

Address Negative Thoughts: Those with low self-worth often allow negative self-talk to impact their mood and confidence. But thoughts are not always reality, so face those thoughts and replace them with factual statements of affirmation.

Search Out Support: People without a strong sense of worth often live their entire lives that way, but the thought process can have an increasingly detrimental effect on one's relationships, career, and overall happiness. A therapist can provide the support you need to relearn thought processes and gradually boost your self-worth.

If you think you have low self-esteem and that the mindset is adversely affecting your life, you can take proactive steps to improve your situation. Respecting and valuing yourself can be a meaningful step toward finding the respect and consideration of others.

Keeping a commitment or a promise is a major deposit; breaking one is a major withdrawal. People tend to build their hopes around promises, particularly promises about their basic livelihood.

—*The 7 Habits of Highly Effective People*
by Stephen Covey

Chapter 13

The Importance of Honoring Commitments

If someone routinely breaks promises, they may not think it matters. But honoring commitments (or failing to do so) significantly impacts our relationships and our feelings. While it seems a lofty concept, honoring commitments can be defined simply: You do what you said you were going to do, and you do it when you said you would. The ramifications of failing to honor a commitment are serious, whether those commitments are life-changing (promising financial support) or trivial (assuring someone you will call them back). But the ramifications of failing to honor a commitment, no matter how small, is more serious than we think. Each failed commitment tells the subconscious mind that you are not a trustworthy person. To the world at large, you are someone whose word cannot be trusted or relied upon. It does not take long before people lose respect for someone who fails to honor their commitments. Perhaps more devastating is the loss of self-respect that can take place. The good news is that the opposite is just as powerful—honoring your commitments gives meaning and weight to your words.

Psychologically Speaking

When you make a commitment and then back out of it, what you're really saying is "My time and my choices are more valuable than yours." Of course, there are emergencies that justify failing to come through, but true emergencies are pretty rare.

Not long after I went into practice, I realized it was essential to have a cancellation/no show fee. Clients would routinely schedule an appointment, filling up my schedule, then cancel because they had something else they had to attend. I found it very disheartening when the blame was placed back on me for not being understanding and flexible.

Call To Action

If you find you have trouble honoring commitments, here are a few tips:

Practice Saying "No": One sure way to protect your integrity is to limit those things you commit to. In other words, learn to say no. Many people have a problem refusing a request but then find it challenging to juggle everything they have agreed to do. When we say yes to things that do not align with our priorities, we create a self-imposed situation wherein we are tempted to back out. By identifying those things you wish to participate in, you can politely turn down those requests that do not align with your priorities.

Honor Self-Commitments: If we don't even honor our commitments to ourselves, we are unlikely to honor those we make with others. Start by limiting the number of things on your personal to-do list, then make sure you accomplish them. You can always add more to the list as you grow in discipline.

Another great way to honor commitments is to be realistic and make promises to yourself slowly. If you wish to change your diet, don't give up everything at once—concentrate on one thing at a time. If you want to begin exercising, start with a manageable regimen. Don't try to run ten miles on the first day. Making and honoring realistic commitments to yourself teaches your brain that you can change your behavior.

Honor Commitments to Others: Just as learning to honor commitments to yourself is imperative, keeping promises we make to others is necessary for good mental health and robust relationships. You may not think you break commitments often, but this happens every day in many ways.

- You promise to run an errand for someone but then don't do it, saying "I don't have enough time."
- You say you'll provide information or feedback by a specific date or time but fail to do so.
- You don't show up for a scheduled appointment, whether with a dentist or hair stylist.

When you don't honor your commitments to others, it won't be long before people don't trust what you say, lose respect for you, or consider you unreliable. However, when you begin to honor your commitments, great and small, you develop a sense of control over your life. You transform yourself into the kind of person who does what you promise. You begin to feel pride and respect, a worthwhile goal for anyone.

Between stimulus and response, there is
a space. In that space lies our freedom
and power to choose our response. In our
response lies our growth and freedom.

—*Viktor Frankl*

Chapter 14

The Importance of Emotional Intelligence

Most of us have heard of the intelligence quotient, or IQ, which measures one's cognitive learning abilities. But perhaps more important is a person's emotional intelligence (EQ or EI), which is how well an individual responds emotionally to situations. Emotional intelligence is characterized by the level of empathy and understanding a person has, not by their educational excellence. How important is EQ to navigating life?

Emotional intelligence is vital to forming and maintaining close, healthy personal relationships. While our cognitive intelligence remains essentially the same throughout our lifetime, EQ can—and does—increase with our desire to pursue emotional growth. Characteristics of high EQ individuals include:

- **Independence**—they are self-controlled and self-directed.

- **Self-actualization**—they reach for their true potential.

- **Self-awareness**—they recognize their own emotions and the effects of their reactions on others.

- **Impulse control**—they resist impulses to act inappropriately.

- **Flexibility**—they adapt their emotions to changing situations.

- **Resilience**—they look at life optimistically and keep a positive outlook in adverse circumstances.

- **Social responsibility**—they cooperate and contribute to society while maintaining responsibility, honesty, and integrity.

- **Empathy**—they understand and exhibit awareness of the feelings of others.

- **Stress tolerance**—they withstand adverse events without "falling apart."

- **Problem solving**—they identify problems and implement effective solutions.

- **Assertiveness**—they confidently communicate beliefs, emotions, and thoughts in a non-destructive manner.

Psychologically Speaking

I have seen the brightest of human beings struggle with a low EQ. While our logical brain might easily recall facts, logic, and data, it is our emotional intelligence that helps us with timing, awareness, and empathy. I have found that a low EQ is the most noticeable when people communicate. For example, you begin telling a story at a dinner party, but it is obvious by the body language of the other guests that they are either not interested or offended. Yet, you keep on telling the story. Accepting the "no" of others when they don't want to talk or don't want to buy what you're selling is an example of a higher EQ.

Call to Action

Emotionally intelligent people have more success navigating life, coping with stress, and maintaining life-giving relationships, so achieving a higher EQ is desirable for all of us.

Here are some tips to do just that:

Minimize Negative Emotions: People cannot change their reactions unless they change their emotions and perspective. This is done primarily by avoiding jumping to conclusions and considering alternative explanations for a given situation. For instance, instead of feeling rejected because someone didn't return your text, remind yourself that they are likely otherwise engaged and will answer when they can. Individuals can also avoid feelings of rejection by expanding their alternatives. For example, instead of relying on one job opportunity, apply for a wide range of jobs that interest you.

Stay Cool in the Face of Stress: When faced with stress, you have a choice—you can be calm and poised or lose your cool. Those who wish to raise EQ should work to dissipate their nervous emotions when they feel stressed, perhaps by stopping to pray, taking a walk outside, or listening to an upbeat song. More intense physical activity may be warranted if the situation inspires fear or depression. A famous adage states that "motion dictates emotion." The more physically active an individual is, the more confidence they will have in stressful situations.

Express Tough Emotions: Everyone needs to set appropriate boundaries, which includes advocating for their right to disagree, saying "no" without guilt, setting personal priorities, and protecting themselves from harm. Individuals can achieve this by learning to express themselves using the XYZ technique, stating, "I feel X when you do Y in situation Z. " Practically speaking, this may sound like:

I feel disappointed when you don't do what you promised you would do.

I feel taken advantage of when you ask me to do something without giving me any notice.

I feel dismissed when you refuse to listen to my opinion.

People should avoid "you" language that may make the listener defensive when expressing themselves, e.g., "You never follow through on a promise."

Remain Proactive, Not Reactive: Everyone has unreasonable people in their work or personal life, and all too often, they let them ruin their mood or, worse, their entire day. People with a high EQ take a proactive approach to interactions with these people, taking a deep breath and waiting before responding to let the immediate reaction pass. Another method to dealing with difficult people is to learn more about what may be causing them to be so unpleasant—to feel empathy for them rather than annoyance. For instance, if they are a caregiver for a sick parent or have recently lost a spouse, you can better understand the source of their anger and frustration. While empathy does not excuse their bad behavior, it reminds us that the issue resides with them and not with the target of their emotions.

Show Resilience in Adversity: Everyone faces adversity to one degree or another, but those with a high EQ have learned to think, feel, and act in such a way that they experience hope instead of despair, optimism instead of pessimism, and victory versus defeat. They react to a difficult situation with the question "How can I learn from this experience?" rather than "Why do these things always happen to me?" The quality of the questions that we ask dictates our outcome. Constructive questions prioritize learning and perspective rather than victimhood and distress.

Express Intimate Emotions: The ability and willingness to both express and validate loving emotions is vital to cultivating close relationships. Sharing intimate feelings in a healthy and constructive manner—and responding affirmatively to the other party's expression of the same—results from high EQ development. Loving words and actions can manifest in a million ways, all of which relate that the parties to the relationship care about each other and value the other's presence in their life.

Every day we have plenty of opportunities to get angry, stressed, or offended. But what you're doing when you indulge these negative emotions is giving something outside yourself power over your happiness. You can choose to not let little things upset you.

—*Joel Osteen*

Chapter 15

Anger

Everyone gets angry occasionally. It is typically a quick reaction we resort to when we need to let off steam. But sometimes anger manifests in ways that are irrational or over the top. When unchecked, anger can have a significant impact on your life, your health, and your personal relationships. It is important to be aware of proactive ways for diffusing anger and de-escalating the situation.

Here are a few helpful ways to diffuse anger before acting out.

1. Think about it: We've all been told to "count to ten" when we want to lash out in anger, and the advice is sound. When we are upset, it is easy to say something we will later regret. Take the time you need—ten seconds or ten minutes—to calm down and think through your reaction.

2. Speak your concerns when you are calm: Once thoughts have cleared, communicate your frustration in a non-confrontational but confident way. Identify your worries and offenses without harming others or trying to manipulate them.

3. Think more about solutions: Instead of obsessing about the object of your anger, put your efforts toward a resolution and a solution to the problem. Begin to accept that some things are not yours to control, change, or fix. Remind yourself that reacting in anger won't resolve anything—and may aggravate the situation.

4. Take a deep breath: When anger starts to take control, relaxation skills such as deep-breathing exercises can help tremendously to diffuse the emotion. You may choose to imagine a favorite place in nature, repeat a calming mantra, listen to music, or stretch out into a few yoga poses.

Psychologically Speaking

Yelling, anger, and rage are ways to blow off steam and get rid of excess tension in the body. And while it may be appropriate to yell if you are walking down the street and see someone stepping off the curb into the path of an oncoming bus, in most situations it is inappropriate and ineffective.

And it's not just bad for the recipient of the anger. The body doesn't know what situations are real or imagined. It relies on the mind to cue it so it can appropriately respond. Whenever a person yells or becomes overly heated in a situation, the body releases stress hormones, which can cause a lot of strain on the heart. Heart attacks, lung problems, high blood pressure, and breast issues in women are just a few ways the body can manifest physical problems as a result of this excess strain on the heart.

Call to Action

When you address any situation, make sure you honor the other person and, most of all, honor yourself. All situations can be handled with ease, addressed clearly, and without heightened emotions. We don't need to be hostile or disrespectful to make a point.

Because people don't deal with fear objectively, they don't understand it. They end up keeping their fear and trying to prevent things from happening that would stimulate it. They go through life attempting to create safety and control by defining how they need life to be in order to be okay. This is how the world becomes frightening.

—*The Untethered Soul*
by Michael A. Singer

Chapter 16

How to Recognize If You Are A "People Pleaser"

A people pleaser is an individual who routinely puts others' needs ahead of their own. This type of person is highly sensitive to those around them and can be considered helpful, kind, and gracious. At first, the traits of a people pleaser can seem admirable and noble. And why not? The world can be a difficult place, and we could all use a little more kindness and generosity. Unfortunately, people pleasers rarely know how to advocate for themselves, neglecting their own needs and falling into a harmful cycle of self-neglect and self-sacrifice. This pattern is due to a personality trait known as "sociotropy." These individuals become overly concerned with pleasing others and think the only way to maintain their relationships is by earning others' approval.

People pleasers tend to exhibit the following traits:

- Difficulty saying no—or feeling guilty about saying no

- Being overly worried about what people think
- Having the belief that turning people down will appear mean or selfish
- Having low self-esteem
- Wanting to be liked, doing things for people to earn approval
- Always apologizing
- Taking the blame no matter the circumstance
- Never having free time because of commitments to other people.

Psychologically Speaking

We may think a people pleaser is motivated to help or please others. But in reality, people pleasers are pleasing to relieve their own anxiety and fear. It is a symptom of low self-esteem, poor boundaries, guilt, and anxiety.

So what can you do if you are a people pleaser? When someone is unhappy or something needs to be taken care of, take a moment and learn more about the situation by asking questions. Not only will this help you clarify the situation, it will also give you time to create space and allow your anxious energy to clear some. Do your best to resist rushing in and rescuing. If you are a spiritual person, it may be helpful to understand that God or the Universe teaches through pain, discomfort, and often disappointment. If we didn't feel discomfort, we would never pay attention to situations or experiences. There are always lessons and growth opportunities in setbacks. Be mindful of when helping is appropriate and when it is harmful. I would be happy to help you learn more.

Call to Action

Fear is a low vibrational yet intense emotion that often caus-es us to act impulsively and inappropriately. Fear is the tool of the ego and will lead us to believe we need to get involved. Allow fear to come up, process it, and then let it pass. If the fear is present in a dangerous situation, there may not be many options available. But most of the things we fear are perceived or imag-ined. You may feel comfort just knowing that.

By keeping the end clearly in mind, you can make certain that whatever you do on any particular day does not violate the criteria you have defined as supremely important, and that each day of your life contributes in a meaningful way to the vision you have of your life as a whole.

—*The 7 Habits of Highly Effective People*
by Stephen Covey

Chapter 17

Fighting Procrastination

Procrastination is an exercise of unnecessary delay. People prone to procrastination understand that the delay or postponement is not beneficial, but they do it anyway. Overcoming procrastination is possible through self-care and setting goals.

Many people who procrastinate feel as if they are the only ones who pay the price. Yet procrastination is not a harmless act. It keeps you from accomplishing more important, meaningful tasks, leading you instead to trivial activities with little value. Chronic procrastination can lead to mental and physical health issues, impact our financial well-being, and even sabotage academic or career goals. Those who procrastinate experience elevated stress levels and can live with depression, anxiety, or cardiovascular disease.

While not scientifically categorized, mental health experts have identified these types of attitudes behind the behavior:

- **It's Got to Be Perfect:** The perfectionist will constantly criticize their own work, generally fearing failure. The very high standards they hold for themselves cause anxiety and stress relating to what needs to be done.

- **I've Got Plenty of Time:** When people believe that there is still ample time remaining before the task's deadline, they will put it off until the very last minute.

- **I'm So Bored:** When people think their necessary work is mundane, they will often look for other things to do that they consider more fun.

- **This Stresses Me Out:** When tasks inspire anxiety or stress, someone may procrastinate as a coping mechanism. However, this situation is a catch-22 because the longer the task is delayed, the more anxious they become.

Psychologically Speaking

Researchers believe that people allow the desire for instant gratification to divert them from demanding tasks or goals. Procrastinating is a short-term mood-regulation strategy that has long-term consequences and results from several emotional variables, including:

- Depression, stress, or anxiety
- Fatigue or lack of energy
- High blood pressure and cardiovascular disease
- Low self-esteem, regret, and loss of satisfaction in their life

Call to Action

Here are some strategies to help avoid procrastination:

1. **Future Self vs. Present Self:** Many people go to sleep each evening with a long list of what they plan to achieve the next day, but when the morning arrives,

their motivation vanishes. This is because, for many, planning for the future is significantly easier than tackling short-term goals. Visualizing yourself completing the activity and the benefits you will reap from that achievement can bring the future and present together. Picturing success also allows us to focus on priorities when setting the schedule for the day.

2. **Closely Held Deadlines:** Research proves that having less time makes people more productive. Maintaining tight deadlines for every task—and putting everything into a schedule and a calendar—motivates people to accomplish things on time. Not achieving personal daily deadlines may cause guilt and shame, which, although unpleasant, can be a great motivator.

3. **Schedule Your Breaks:** Procrastination studies prove that we will avoid working on complex or tedious tasks to fill the time with something more attractive. Scheduling breaks provides a respite we can look forward to and ultimately improves productivity when we return to the task. Breaks for personal time may include outdoor walks, meeting someone for a meal, or indulging in a favorite pastime.

4. **Set Practical Limits:** Those whose work involves the computer often find themselves wasting time on social media or surfing the internet. Others may turn on the TV "for just a few minutes." Procrastinators can allow themselves these guilty pleasures as long as they are regulated by strict time frames (such as allowing five minutes at the top of each hour to check their social accounts.) Tracking activities in a time journal can help with accountability.

5. **Offer Yourself Compassion and Grace:** Negative emotions often contribute to procrastination, leading to more negative emotions. It's a complicated cycle that is difficult to escape and can devastate self-esteem. The guilt that results from chronic delaying can be alleviated by forgiving yourself and accepting that you are struggling. Acknowledging the difficulty you are experiencing opens the door to accepting grace and inspiring future motivation to do better.

A borderline suffers a kind of emotional hemophilia; they lack the clotting mechanism needed to moderate spurts of feelings. Stimulate a passion, and the borderline emotionally will bleed to death.

—*I Hate You–Don't Leave Me*
by Hal Straus and Jerold Jay Kreisman

Chapter 18

Borderline Personality Disorder

Borderline personality disorder is a mental health condition that impacts how individuals think and feel about themselves and the people around them. The disorder may cause a person to struggle with self-worth and have difficulty maintaining authentic relationships and managing emotions.

Those with borderline personality disorder fear abandonment and often can't cope with feeling alone or isolated, resulting in inappropriate bursts of anger, impulsiveness, and volatile mood swings. These emotions can make it difficult for a person with borderline personality disorder to form healthy relationships.

The onset of borderline personality disorder typically occurs in early adulthood, when the symptoms are most pronounced. As the individual ages, the effects may gradually decrease. But there is no need to wait until the disorder fades on its own. With proper attention and treatment, a person can lead a full and engaging life.

Psychologically Speaking

Borderline personality disorder cannot be officially diagnosed until a person turns eighteen, but many children and adolescents show behavioral traits early on.

These types of mental health disorders impact how people feels about themselves and how they behave around others. Possible clues that you or a loved one may be experiencing borderline personality disorder include:

- An overwhelming fear of abandonment that causes the individual to pursue radical measures to avoid separation or rejection.

- A series of unstable and volatile relationships, with emotions often swinging quickly from putting someone on a pedestal to thinking they are mean or insensitive.

- Changes in self-identity and self-esteem that occur rapidly and cause individuals to adjust their values, often viewing themselves as invisible or even "bad."

- Continued and extended sense of loneliness and emptiness.

- Dangerous and impulsive behavior that can cause self-harm, such as spending sprees, reckless driving, casual/unsafe sex, binge eating, gambling, or drug abuse.

- Sabotages quality of life and success by quitting a good job or terminating a positive relationship abruptly and for no good reason.

- Threats of suicide or self-injury often related to the fear of rejection or separation.

- Violent mood swings, which can involve waves of deep happiness followed by intense irritability or overwhelming shame or anxiety.

- Intense and inappropriate rages that may include engaging in physical fights.

Call To Action

If you've become aware of any of the signs listed above, it is best to speak with your physician or a mental health counselor. This is essential if the behaviors have recently developed, have a negative impact on your job, or adversely affect core relationships.

Are You Suicidal? Anyone experiencing thoughts or fantasies of suicide or self-harm, do not delay taking proactive action.

- Call 911 or a suicide hotline immediately. In the United States, call or text 988 to reach the 988 Suicide & Crisis Lifeline, available twenty-four hours a day, seven days a week. Or use the Lifeline Chat. Services are free and confidential.

- Contact your physician or mental health provider.

> A lack of boundaries invites a lack of respect.
>
> —*Author unknown*

Chapter 19

Setting and Enforcing Boundaries

Boundaries are rules and limits an individual creates to set reasonable, permissible, and safe ways for others to interact with them. They also set guidelines that outline an acceptable response when someone violates those limits. Boundaries are personal "property lines" no one can cross without consequence, although they can be challenging because they can't be seen and are unique to every individual.

Personal boundaries determine the amount of physical and emotional space someone allows between themselves and others. They define what levels of communication and interaction are acceptable and what behaviors are tolerable.

There are many reasons people choose to establish boundaries for themselves.

- To practice self-care
- To cultivate self-respect
- To effectively communicate relational needs
- To allow space for more positive interactions

Setting boundaries is a key component to our physical and emotional health. Unhealthy or inappropriate boundaries can result in emotional pain, codependency, anxiety, depression, and even stress-related disease. Without healthy boundaries, anyone can intrude on your life at any time. Some people have difficulty trusting themselves and then put up a very thick boundary around themselves. However, building too thick of a wall can result in isolation and loneliness, which can be just as unhealthy. It can be hard for others to connect to us if we don't allow them to be a part of our lives in a healthy manner.

Psychologically Speaking

Most people understand which behaviors trigger their emotional or physical responses and can quickly identify the boundaries they want to put into place, but few are comfortable with enforcing or upholding their own rules. The most common reasons for this are:

- Fear of rejection and abandonment
- Fear of confrontation
- Guilt about setting rules for others

When establishing guidelines, individuals should be clear, firm, and respectful. There is no need to justify the boundary, nor is there a reason to apologize. Apologizing sends a mixed message to those with whom you are communicating. You are responsible for communicating the boundary respectfully, but you are not responsible for the other person's reaction. If you tend to become defensive, over-explain, or become heated when communicating what you want, you might benefit from some professional help understanding boundaries more clearly.

Call to Action

Get out a piece of paper and make a large circle. Inside the circle, write a few words that describe your values. For example, "honesty from myself and others." Respect for myself and others." Be honest with yourself about your true values. Are they values you have been living? Would others recognize your description of yourself? I have had many incidents, in sessions, where the client had very little or no self-awareness.

After you are comfortable with what you have written in your circle, think about whether or not the people and circumstances in your life align with what you have defined as important. For example, if you described yourself as a kind person, spending time around negative friends who enjoy talking badly about others might not be right for you.

Nobody can be kinder than a narcissist
while you react to life on his terms.

—*Elizabeth Bowen*

Chapter 20

Understanding Narcissistic Personality Disorders

The term "narcissist" has become popular in our world today and is often overutilized to describe people we simply don't like. But someone who is overly confident or even selfish is not necessarily a narcissist, even if they may be unpopular. In its truest form, narcissism is a personality disorder marked by evident characteristics.

The following nine traits are used to define a narcissist, and at least five must be present for the disorder to be diagnosed.

1. **Grandiose self-importance:** Narcissists often believe that their presence is essential for the happiness of the people in their life or the success of a business project.

   Characteristic statement: *They would be nothing without me.*

2. **Preoccupation with thoughts of unlimited success, power, intelligence, or beauty:** A narcissist may believe that they can achieve extraordinary

things even when there is no accurate indication that these things are possible.

Characteristic statement: *Even though I'm entry-level now, I should be in management within six months—I already know more than my boss!*

3. **Belief that they are unique and better than others:** Narcissists believe that they should be able to talk with a top-level person in any situation and often name-drop to make themselves seem more influential than they really are.

Characteristic statement: *I don't deal with anyone but the company owner—they know me by name.*

4. **Need for excessive admiration:** The narcissist isn't looking for acknowledgment or a pat on the back; they seek esteem and honor over and above normal levels. They may "fish for compliments" until others comment on and admire their looks, clothes, or accomplishments. Bragging is natural for narcissists as well.

Characteristic statement: *Don't you love how I look in this outfit?*

5. **Sense of entitlement:** Narcissists believe they deserve the best jobs, the nicest car, or the best seat at the ballgame, and their actions and achievements are often out of line with their sense of entitlement.

Characteristic statement: *That promotion belonged to me! I deserved it more than he did.*

6. **Behavior that exploits relationships:** Narcissists see other people as a means to an end, exhibiting a lack of awareness that other individuals have desires, emotions, and goals of their own. Whatever they

pursue is to further their own interest—and they expect others to move out of the way for them. If others suffer or lose out, it does not bother them.

Characteristic statement: *"Get out of my way! I'm in a hurry!"*

7. **Lack of empathy:** Narcissists lack the emotional awareness to appropriately recognize how other people feel. Contrary to popular belief, it is not that narcissists don't "care" about someone's feelings; it is more that they are completely unaware that other people even have those feelings at all.

Characteristic statement: *"They don't mind that I took their place; they know I deserve it."*

8. **Belief that others are envious of them:** Narcissists constantly compare themselves to others and believe that everyone around them is jealous of their stature. Being considered "ordinary" or "typical" would be a massive blow to their ego, one they could not accept.

Characteristic statement: *"Everyone looks to me for advice and guidance."*

9. **Demonstration of arrogant attitudes:** Conceit and arrogance are often the first things you notice about a narcissist. They will expect—or even demand—that others act as they want them to. While this is often evidenced in condescending statements, the behavior may also manifest in confident or rude actions, such as placing themselves at the front of a line.

Characteristic statement: *We can go to counseling together to prove that you're the problem.*

Psychologically Speaking

A person with narcissistic personality disorder rarely comes to my office. As you can imagine, a person who feels they are superior to others or they "know it all" would not be the type of person who would come in for counseling and allow themselves to be vulnerable. However, it is not unusual for me to see this type of personality in marriage or couples counseling. A person with narcissistic personality traits will only partner with someone who allows for or accommodates their tendencies. In rare instances, one of these individuals will convince the other that a therapist might be able to help.

What I have heard from the narcissistic individual many times is "I felt it was important to come in so that you could tell my wife she is wrong." As you can imagine, this type of session can be extremely difficult to navigate. On average, I usually only see this type of case for three or four sessions before the narcissistic partner makes the dependent partner feel guilty or one of them (sometimes both of them) get upset with me and cancel all their future appointments.

Call to Action

If you are in a relationship with a narcissist, you probably feel trapped. But remember, you are not a victim and you do have choices. If you are not willing to get out of the relationship, you must learn to live with your partner and accept things the way they are. Things will not likely change. If you feel like you are slowly suffocating and want to start your life over, happier and healthier, you have to muster the courage to leave.

Remember, a narcissist is a master manipulator and it may not be easy, but it is possible. Narcissists always need to feel in power and have control. A domestic help hotline can offer help and assistance.

One day you will tell your story of how you overcame what you went through and it will be someone else's survival guide.

—Amazingmemovement.com

Chapter 21

How Past Trauma Affects Your Life

Everyone will experience some type of trauma in their lifetime. Trauma can occur from a range of experiences, from military combat to the death of a pet. The degree to which trauma affects someone's life can vary greatly. Many experience a numbing sensation when they are faced with trauma, and they focus on extraneous details rather than the source of their trauma. For example, the sudden death of a family member can put a person into overdrive as they get busy planning the funeral, hosting family, and breezing through life on what appears to be pure adrenaline.

People view trauma differently. I have had clients say the death of a pet was very traumatic for them. Other clients have described horrific abuse, almost too overwhelming to hear, but they do not seem traumatized. Which reminds me that trauma is a lot like what I learned about pain in nursing school. Pain is what the patient says it is. Trauma is no different. It is important to honor both ourselves and others when tragedy and suffering come our way.

Psychologically Speaking

Unfortunately, we cannot escape trauma and all the pain and emotions that come along with it. The challenge and harmful effects arise when we hold trauma in our bodies. After months or even years of holding trauma, it is not unusual for people to suffer from physical conditions. Back pain is a common way the body responds to trauma. I have also seen many clients struggle with other chronic pain, autoimmune disorders, and even cancer.

If you are struggling with something that happened to you in the past, give yourself the gift of healing. It may be hard to imagine, but sometimes good things happen as a result of something bad happening. Psychological changes after trauma are possible when individuals acknowledge their struggles and identify more as survivors than victims. These people build resilience, learn practical coping skills, and develop a sense of self-sufficiency. They may experience more long-lasting relationships, find a new spiritual purpose, or cultivate a more meaningful appreciation for life.

Call to Action

This may seem impossible, but when the body experiences trauma or even an overwhelming emotional event, self-care is essential. Many of us feel guilty taking care of ourselves because they feel it is important to suffer as a result of what they experienced. Think about it this way: after we have surgery or a procedure, the doctor prescribes rest and self-care. With emotional trauma, the recommendation is the same. Self-care can include things like walking to the mailbox, sitting outside in the sunshine, taking a hot bath, praying, attending a religious service, meditating. Have compassion on the body and allow it to heal. Remember, it is not "if" you heal but "how" you heal that is important. A therapist or counselor can also help.

Today's thought came from a dear friend of mine who texted me when I was grieving a painful loss. She had lost her son when he was only sixteen and was more than familiar with grief. She said, "All emotions must be felt and dealt with in order to get to the other side and move forward. And it moves at its own pace. There is no need to spend energy trying to rush it because it doesn't work that way."

—*Irmelin Toftegaard*

Chapter 22

Understanding and Coping with Grief

As natural as grief is, it is one of the most difficult emotions to process and understand. There are many misconceptions surrounding grief, including what it should look like and how long it should last. There is no "right or wrong" or appropriate way to grieve. A person's experience with profound sadness depends on many factors, such as personality, life experience, faith or belief system, and the significance of the loss.

Although grief is unpleasant, and you may want it over quickly, healing is a gradual process that plays an important role. You cannot force or hurry emotions along. While some people begin to feel better in a few weeks or several months, others experience grief for years. The most important thing to remember is that there is no set time frame for grieving.

When we think of grief, we may associate it with the most intense type of grief after losing a loved one, but many situations in life may cause these emotions.

- Divorce or the breakup of a relationship, loss of a friendship

- Miscarriage
- Retirement, loss of a job, or loss of financial stability
- Personal illness or illness of a loved one
- The death of a pet
- Selling a longtime family home
- Unfulfilled dreams
- Loss of security or safety after a traumatic event

Psychologically Speaking

Many people who are grieving get stuck in the "waiting room." They know their life will never be the same, but they have no idea how to move forward into their new life. The thought of it can cause extreme anxiety and fear. This is why self-care is essential to help the body, mind, and soul heal.

One of the medical approaches to grief I sometimes struggle with is treating grief with medication. This may be helpful in some instances, but I don't recommend rushing into it, as grief can be a wonderful teacher. It gives us a time to pause and reflect on the things we appreciate and also offers an opportunity for those who love us to support us.

Call to Action

When we have a surgical procedure, extra self-care is essential for a successful recovery and optimal healing. We are usually compliant with doctor's orders because we generally are in pain and want to heal as quickly as possible. Grief and emotional pain are no different. When we are grieving, it is important to give ourselves a lot of self-care, compassion, and grace. I will offer a few suggestions, but it is important that you decide what feels right for you. For example, a hot bath will not be beneficial if you don't like taking baths.

Suggestions for self-care and healing:

- Taking a walk with a friend.

- Journaling about your feelings and things you are grateful for at the end of each day.

- Using calming aromatherapy, such as lavender.

- Ensuring you are eating regularly and drinking plenty of water.

- Resting or taking a nap if you are feeling exhausted.

- Resisting the need to answer every text and phone call, or to host company if you are not up to it.

- Tuning into your body and giving it what it needs.

- Getting help from a therapist, either in person or virtually. Self-scheduling is easy on my website at *deniseschonwald.com.*

All emotions are neutral. They have no
meaning other than the meaning we assign
to them. An emotion is like a burst
of energy that quickly circulates around
the mind and body, indicating that there
is an imbalance that needs to be brought
into balance. The moment you experience a
burst of emotionally charged energy,
suspend all judgment of yourself for
whatever it is and ride it out.

—*Iyanla Van Zant*

Chapter 23

Effects of Chronic Stress on Body and Mind

Today's world presents us with many challenging situations. The fast pace of life and the relentless news cycle is causing chronic stress for many people, which can adversely affect the mind and body. Because the nervous system cannot differentiate between physical and emotional threats, the body may react just as strongly to an argument with a good friend as to a car accident.

Someone who experiences frequent stress constantly lives in a heightened state of anxiety, which can result in serious health issues. Chronic stress disrupts nearly every functional system in the body, including the immune, digestive, and reproductive systems. Stress can even rewire the brain, making the individual more susceptible to anxiety, depression, and other mental conditions.

Psychologically Speaking

Living in a world that is unpredictable and challenging at times can be both exciting and scary. We not only experience our own emotions but we also take on the emotions and feelings of those we spend time with. For example, you could walk into a funeral home and visit with the family of the deceased, perhaps a friend of a friend, and later leave exhausted. The stress of a situation could have an impact on you, regardless of whether it was personal to you or not.

Even if we are having a great day, meeting clients or friends, it can be tiring. Stress in our mind comes from situations, real or imagined, which can eventually manifest physically. If we are irrational thinkers, the mind has to use a lot of energy. You may notice that if your mind is really active, you eat more sweets and carbohydrates. This is because the mind needs a lot of fuel to do its thing, and both sugar and carbs convert to energy quickly. Alcohol also has a lot of sugar and even though we hope it will help us relax, it actually just provides temporary relief and can be a slippery slope to attachment or addiction if we are not careful.

Here are some ways to manage stress:

1. **Turn Off the Screens:** Because of mobile devices, we are "at work" even while sitting at home—an even greater reality for those who are remote employees. Checking and responding to emails from the phone can easily rob us of time that should be spent with kids at the park or disrupt time with a spouse or friends at dinner. All those lights and stimuli also trigger the brain to work harder and prevent relaxation or rest. So turn off the screens for a few hours each day and relax with your loved ones.

2. **Just Say No:** Somewhere along the line, overcommitment became a virtue, but it is detrimental to a balanced life. Learning to say "no" once in a while is

incredibly freeing and allows you to regain control over your free time. Say yes only when the request represents an activity that is essential, valuable, or brings you joy.

3. **Be Diligent about Your Health:** Maintaining a vibrant quality of life is difficult when you feel sick, exhausted, or in pain. Your body will tell you when your life is out of balance. Maximum productivity and happiness result from adequate sleep, healthy eating, and physical activity. It all starts with getting enough rest. Without sleep, you will feel tired, experience brain fog, and feel your motivation drop.

4. **Reduce Toxic Influence:** It really is true—people who engage in toxic behaviors can steal your joy, distract you, negatively impact your productivity, and cause you to lie awake at night. While it is impossible to avoid whiners, complainers, and narcissists all the time, working to reduce the amount of time spent around them will boost your overall mood.

5. **Spend Time Alone:** These days, scheduling time alone is nearly inconceivable. With your day carved up between career and family—with a few moments with friends thrown in—there isn't a lot of time for a leisurely walk through the woods. However, that walk may be essential for a healthy balance in your life. Time alone reduces stress, boosts well-being, and inspires creativity. Incorporating meditation or prayer can also help you achieve balance and moments of serenity.

6. **But Don't Neglect Relationships:** Conversely, fulfilling social and relational needs is critical for a healthy life. Turn off the devices and genuinely engage with your partner, spouse, or kids. Connect and be present for those you care about.

Call to Action

When the body is not in balance, when you aren't managing stress with rest and play, the body will start to manifest through behaviors. Overeating, drinking, irritability, spending, and smoking are all signs the body needs ease. Make it a practice to check in with yourself and notice how you are feeling throughout the day. If you are not sure, observe how you are acting or how other people appear to be perceiving you. It is easier to make a change or shift sooner rather than later.

...illness not only has a history but also tells a history. It is a culmination of a life-long history of struggle within the self.

—*When the Body Says No*
by Gabor Maté,

Chapter 24

The Emotional Impact of Chronic Disease

Mixed emotions can surface when an individual is diagnosed with a chronic disease. Some types of diseases have no cure—and that means that the individual's life has changed forever.

Chronic diseases like arthritis, IBS, and fibromyalgia can cause recurring pain flare-ups and relapses. These medical conditions can also cause emotional stress, reduce energy levels, and increase mental fatigue, potentially leading to anxiety and depression.

There are many ways that mental health can be compromised when a person is living with a chronic illness. Here are some examples.

1. **Hormones:** Many illnesses affect the body's function by influencing hormones and neurotransmitters. Hormones control emotions and neurotransmitters help to manage moods and stress responses, and mental health changes can result should they become unbalanced.

2. **Social Engagement:** Having a chronic illness can interrupt everyday routines and interfere with daily tasks, some jobs, and leisure activities. Some people with chronic disease may have to miss school or work if their symptoms flare up. These individuals may become increasingly isolated from peers and colleagues, inducing anxiety, stress, and depression.

3. **Empathic Emotions:** It is normal to pick up on the energy of those closest to us. When someone is sick, their loved ones may be scared or worried and inadvertently cause even more negative emotions for the patient. When loved ones react to a diagnosis with excessive emotion, the stress can transfer to the patient, who often wants to ease their loved one's pain. This type of cycle can cause even more stress on their relationship.

Psychologically Speaking

In my first book, I talked about the importance of living a physically, emotionally, and spiritually healthy life. A disease, illness, or symptom develops when energy is blocked inside the body when emotions or experiences aren't processed effectively. A disease or illness does not happen randomly—it evolves or manifests. Clinicians have learned the benefits of understanding the energy patterns or meridians in the body. Acupuncturists refer to this energy as chi. It can be difficult for a person to correct irrational thinking patterns or ineffective coping mechanisms when they have little understanding of how the energy in their body is blocked, ultimately manifesting in physical conditions and illnesses.

Call to Action

Make a list of physical ailments and correlate them with emotional issues based on the book *Healing Your Body By Mastering Your Mind*.

Schedule an appointment with me at *deniseschonwald.com*, and I would be happy to help you.

Learn to live as though you are facing death
at all times, and you'll become bolder
and more open. If you live life fully,
you won't have any last wishes. You will
have lived them every moment.

—*The Untethered Soul*
Michael Alan Singer

Chapter 25

Benefits of Hospice Counseling

My husband is a physician, and over the years he has had to give patients unfortunate biopsy results. Many would say, "This is a really bad time to get cancer." There is never a good time to become ill, certainly not terminally ill. But we can use the time we have left after learning we are terminally ill to prepare. We may take that trip we have always said we would take or make plans to see friends and relatives we haven't seen for a long time.

When a person has received a terminal diagnosis, they are at a higher risk for mental health issues. The thought of physical pain and emotional stress can be overwhelming. By providing support to address patients' physical, emotional, and spiritual needs, mental health hospice counseling can offer significant benefits to patients and their families.

Here are five ways that mental health counseling can facilitate the hospice care journey.

1. **Improved quality of life:** Hospice care is designed to assist patients with pain and symptom management, increasing their quality of life. Counseling

can provide support and help patients cope with the emotional challenges of their illness. Understandably, the thought of impending death creates a lot of fear for most people. But with some help, patients can find genuine contentment, happiness, and peace during their final days.

2. More meaningful relationships with friends and family: When terminally ill patients are also experiencing symptoms of a mental health condition, it can disrupt their closest relationships. Hospice care and counseling professionals often provide the emotional support needed to help families communicate and improve relationships. A hospice care counselor can also work with families and friends to prepare them for their loved one's death. Allowing people to share their emotions during hospice can help to ensure their grief is easier to process.

3. Fewer physical health complications: When terminally ill patients have emotional balance, they are more likely to accept needed care and support. Because of these factors, they may be able to enjoy their remaining time without additional physical worries and complications.

4. Appropriately controlled mental health symptoms: Some people have mental health issues before their diagnosis, and others develop depression or anxiety once they get the news. Hospice provides mental health counseling and support to help patients cope with all of the challenges of their situation, from cognitive concerns to depression and anxiety. Sometimes it is determined that medication is appropriate for treating the individual mental health symptoms related to these disorders.

5. Increased dedication to care goals: Hospice providers can also assist with making end-of-life decisions that

agree with the patient's wishes, allowing the best and most compassionate quality of care.

Psychologically Speaking

When we or someone we love receives a diagnosis of terminal illness, many feelings bubble up to the surface. Our own personal struggles may release in the body or maybe some old family issues ignite. When I was a critical care nurse, I witnessed all sorts of family conflict play out in the ICU waiting room. Simple decisions were often magnified, which made end-of-life decisions more difficult.

Determining the right time to initiate hospice care can be challenging, although it is often recommended for patients who are not expected to live beyond the next six months. Mental health and palliative care can work together to offer comfort and coping skills to patients and their families during the grieving process.

Call to Action

End-of-life care and decisions can be overwhelming and frightening. Make a list of your intentions through this journey. Examples:

- Agree to the mantra "Throughout this journey, I will practice grace and dignity."
- Make time for self-care.
- Ask for help and don't feel you need to go down this path alone.
- Rest when you need to.
- Eat regularly even if your meals are smaller.
- Drink plenty of water if you can.

When the mind, body and spirit are in alignment, the energy of the Divine will be ignited.

—*Iyanla Van Zant*

Chapter 26

Does Prayer Improve Our Mental Health?

Many therapists shy away from discussing the importance of spirituality or the power of prayer with regard to mental health, but it can be a very effective tool in healing. Engaging in prayer and meditation can help people of all faiths achieve peace and balance by appealing to something greater than themselves. Practices like prayer and meditation can help the body balance and heal.

Differences Between Prayer and Meditation

Prayer and meditation are two distinctly different activities. The most obvious difference is that prayer is an active practice, typically entered into with a goal in mind. Individuals engaged in prayer speak with a deity they have a relationship with and offer praise or thanks while presenting needs or desires. They often ask for assistance with an expectation of a response.

In contrast, meditation does not attempt to find outside answers the way prayer does. Instead, meditation offers the opportunity to create calm from the inside out, focusing not on responses from a higher power, but instead calling upon one's own consciousness for understanding.

While both practices offer many benefits for mental health, here we will focus on how prayer can help an individual seeking relief from mental trauma and distress. Those who have grown up in a religious household are likely accustomed to praying. Whether it is before a meal or for a specific purpose, prayer is a way to connect not only to God but also to each other. Prayer groups, prayer chains, and having a prayer partner are just some examples.

We know that energy is very powerful. Prayer is a means to surrender our problems to our higher power. It is taking our problems and struggles and releasing them, which ultimately can free the body of stress and pain.

Psychologically Speaking

When the body is under stress, the mind will become extremely active, viewing our situation or circumstance illogically and often through a fearful lens. It can be very difficult to stay mentally healthy when we are under a great deal of stress, even though many people feel they can do it. Prayer and other spiritual practices can be essential tools.

A few practices to deepen spirituality are:

- Meditation, prayers, or deep reflection
- Symbolic and meaningful rituals
- Spending time in nature
- Journaling
- Creative pursuits such as cooking, painting, or gardening, which calms the mind.

- Tai chi, yoga, and other forms of controlled and disciplined exercise

Every day I spend time in prayer. I pray for safety, health, and guidance as I begin my day and before I start seeing patients. I also pray for people I know who are sick, suffering, and grieving. Not long ago, I wondered how many people I was naming and decided to write out a list. I wrote down fifty-five names! This included people I have known since childhood, nurses I worked with, friends who have lost children, patients, and family members of my own. For me, prayer benefits the people I pray for but it also reminds me to be grateful for all the wonderful things in my life.

For me personally, it is comforting to know that I cannot, and do not, need to control or solve all of life's problems. My mom used to say, "Well, I guess you will need to give it to God" when I felt conflicted about a problem in my life. It makes me smile to think how often I remember those words of wisdom from my mom. It brings me a sense of peace to know I am not alone. I hope it brings you peace too.

Call to Action

If you have never incorporated prayer into your daily life, I highly recommend it. Here are a few suggestions to get started:

1. Pray every morning for safety, guidance, and wisdom throughout the day.
2. Pray for your family and friends.
3. Pray before every meal, even if it is a short "thank you for this food" prayer.

4. Pray for those you meet and know are struggling. Make an effort to reach out to them too.

5. Pray that you are able to learn and gain wisdom from your personal setbacks and poor choices.

6. Pray for our country and our leaders, regardless of whether you agree with their politics or not.

7. Pray that the words you speak during the day are kind and thoughtful, particularly when you are disappointed, unhappy, or overwhelmed.

Closing Thoughts

There is so much information available to us today. If we want to learn about something, the internet often provides dozens and dozens of resources, videos, and literature. However, I feel mental health awareness needs to come to the forefront. So many people of all ages and social status struggle with anxiety, depression, or trauma and are not at peace. My hope is that this book can help others gain awareness and ultimately take the next step toward healing.

Asking for help and seeing a therapist is not a sign of weakness. It does not mean you have failed at something or are "less than" because you are struggling. It simply means you are willing to seek out professional help from someone trained and licensed. You wouldn't think twice about calling your physician if you had a physical problem, so why do we think twice about getting help with a psychological struggle? When we take care of ourselves, everyone in our lives benefits from it.

The truth is, we lead by example. It is very easy to give advice, but it is also important that you walk the walk and take care of yourself. It would be hypocritical to ask others to do things you are not willing to do. As a therapist, I work on my own personal growth. I don't "find" time to do it, I "make" time to do it. It is as routine for me as brushing my teeth or taking a shower. I choose to make time for exercise, meditation, journaling, prayer, and counseling when I need it.

Remember, the mind does what you tell it to do. If you say "I choose to take care of myself because I'm worth it," your mind will be the best assistant you could hire. It will help you flow through your day with ease and less pain, suffering, and stress. Our perception is our reality. Make the choice to help others by first helping yourself.

Acknowledgments

I could not be successful without the help of those who work tirelessly right beside me:

Cindy Cunningham has worked with my husband and me for over fifteen years, and I am thankful she stayed on to help me after my husband closed his practice in 2020. She is invaluable to me, taking care of my schedule, the billing, and everything in between.

Chris Williams and his staff at Aginto Digital Marketing came on board this past September, and they have taken the practice to a new level. Chris is always willing to give me the time I need whenever I have a question or a suggestion.

Lastly, my personal assistant Nicole Rodriguez has been invaluable in helping with social media, creating posters, organizing my files, and unscrambling the thoughts in my head.

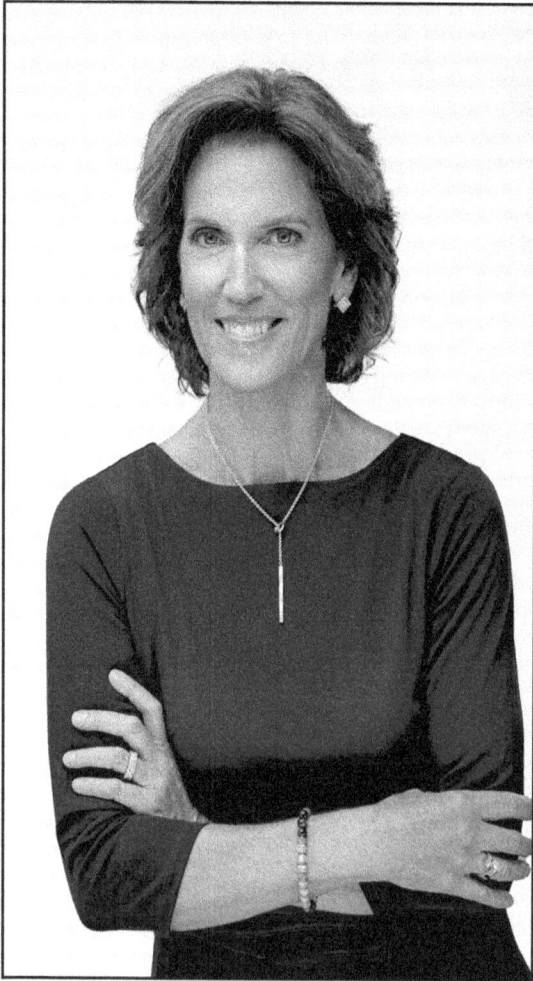

About Denise

In her thirty years working as a registered nurse (BSRN) within the intensive care unit, Denise Schonwald cared for patients who were very ill and often in critical condition. She saw her patients and their families struggling with stress, anxiety, guilt, and fear. She, too, was affected by this challenging environment. In order to help her clients—and herself—cope, Denise learned various techniques to support mental and emotional well-being. Her success in treating the whole person led her to her calling as a spiritually based licensed mental health counselor and mental intuitive (LMHC). By integrating mental health and physical health into a cohesive treatment plan, Denise provides a holistic approach to her patients. These synergistic treatment methodologies support client healing more effectively than traditional counseling.

Denise has expertise in helping clients through a variety of mental and emotional struggles, including anxiety, depression, panic, marital problems, adolescent behavior issues, family issues, childhood trauma, and more. To assist in her method, she draws upon some rather unconventional sources, including Max, a certified therapy dog, who practiced with her until his passing in June of 2020. Henry, his spirited successor, is now her partner in practice. Additional sources of inspiration include physical activity and various forms of meditation, which help relieve stress and provide mental clarity.

Denise personally enjoys boxing, tennis, and yoga, balancing the physical exercise with meditation, Reiki, and aromatherapy to help integrate physical, mental, and spiritual well-being. Understanding the connection between the mind, body, and spirit, Denise helps clients to explore each avenue to achieve optimum levels of health and wellness.

In addition to working with individuals and families, Denise also supports the wider community through speaking engagements and lectures nationwide. Consider having her speak at your next event and contact her office today.

About Henry

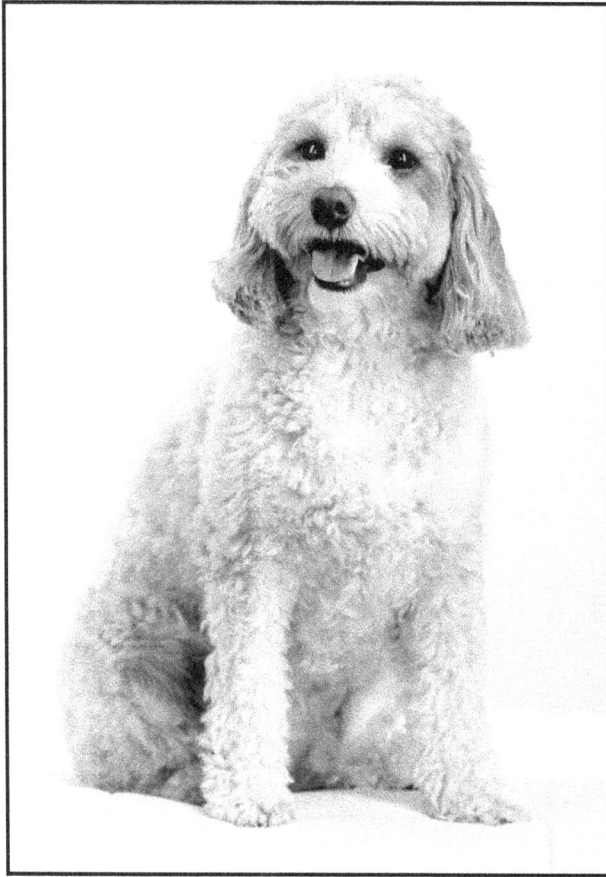

Henry, certified therapy dog, has been practicing with Denise since 2020. He is quite spirited and loves to give hugs to those who have an in-person session. Henry has also been a welcomed guest at Lunch & Learns and other events Denise has lectured.